Dynamic Pulses

Dynamic Pulses

A Brief Introduction to the
Concept of Directionality
and its Reflection of
Organ Function in the Pulses

Ann Cecil-Sterman, MS, L.Ac.

Diagrams by Cody Dodo, MS, L.Ac.

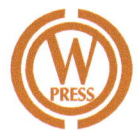

(W) PRESS

Classical
Wellness
Press

First edition

The teachings in this book come from the oral tradition
through the gracious generosity of my principal teacher, Daoist Master, Dr Jeffrey Yuen.
Any mistakes, however, are mine. A.C.S.

Cover design, book design, graphic design and diagrams: Cody Dodo

Front cover calligraphy: "The gentle rains of heaven cleanse us of our illnesses."
Gift of Dr Jeffrey Yuen to the Classical Wellness Center, 2008.

ISBN: 978-0-9837720-4-0

Table of Contents

Acknowledgments

Thanks to **Cody Dodo,** whose unique background as a graphic designer and a Jeffrey Yuen-trained acupuncturist enables him to produce exactly the right diagrams. Thanks for your truly endless patience, expertise, and friendship, Cody. **Andrew Sterman,** who puts his own book authoring and blog aside to read drafts and make corrections. **Betsy Sterman,** for her very detailed, expert corrections and advice on the use of language. **Gretchen Kreiger** for her invaluable and generous support. **Gabrielle Zlotnik, Hope Hathaway, Holly Burling,** for expert proofreading. I appreciate the generosity of **Setareh Moafi** and **Josephine Spilka.** Thank you **Jennifer Jackson** and **Donna Keefe.** Special thanks to **Cissy Majebe** and **Diane Gioioso.**

Introduction

Directional pulse taking is just one of the wide array of pulse techniques. It involves the application and release of pressure from the radial artery. Each organ has one or more vectors: the Stomach's vector is downward, the Spleen's upward, and so on. Directional pulses give a clear reading of whether the organs are operating with their vector intact. For example, if the Spleen's function is not in order, its upward vector may be absent in the pulses. As a guide to the status of the movement of Qi, directional pulses are extremely useful in diagnosis.

Nomenclature

Dynamic Pulses are pulses that require movement of the finger or fingers. Dynamic pulses have two subsets: Probing Pulses and Directional Pulses.

Directional Pulses are pulses that require the application of pressure on one pulse in order to create an effect in another pulse.

Inter-Jiao Blockages are blockages at the diaphragm or in Dai Mai. They obstruct communication between the Jiao's.

Mediumship means any fluid: Jin-Thin Fluids, Ye-Thick Fluids, Blood and Jing-Essence.

Probing Pulses are felt during an inquiry into one individual pulse using varying pressures in that pulse while the pressures applied at the other two positions remain constant.

Pulse Neutral is a term for the basic pulse taking position. The fingers at the cun and guan positions are at the moderate level and the finger at the chi position is at the deep level.

Stepped Position is a term for a pulse taking position where the finger at the cun position is at the superficial level, the finger at the guan position is at the moderate level and the finger at the chi position is at the deep level.

Static Pulses are those that are felt using no movement of the finger once the desired depth is reached.

Bean Classically, Height is said to be measured in beans. The amount of pressure you need to apply for the pulse to yield the required information is measured in the imagined weight of mung beans. This is described in Chapter 5 of the Mai Jing and is figurative, of course. What really matters is the distance your finger travels relative to the total depth of the pulse. The amount of pressure required to press into the bone, occluding the flow of blood in the radial artery, is said to be 15 beans. That is a standard applied to all people, so 15 beans on one person's wrist could be several times the pressure needed on another person's.

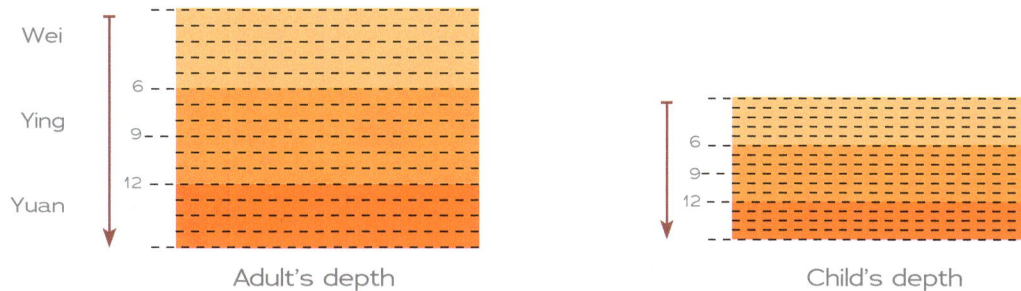

Adult's depth

Child's depth

Part 1

Probing Dynamic Pulses and Organ Function

To understand Dynamic Pulses, it is important to have a clear feeling of the remarkably vast, spacious quality of the pulse. When we first start learning pulses many of us are puzzled that anyone could feel so much detail because the pulses seem such a tiny, shallow part of the anatomy. But the distance we can explore in the pulse is enormously spacious when examined from the surface of the skin down to the level of the bone.

When I teach pulse diagnosis in the classroom, the aspect I need to correct most often is the depth of the fingers at the pulse. When beginning to learn pulse depths, most people think they are deep in the pulse when they are only at about nine beans of pressure. Twelve beans is a long way into the pulse. Fifteen beans requires a considerable pressure.

The following exercise illustrates the surprisingly substantial depth of the pulse. Please take yourself through it before proceeding.

EXERCISE TO EXPERIENCE THE ENTIRE DEPTH EXAMINED IN THE TAKING OF THE PULSE

1. Assume the position of taking the pulses on either your own or a patient's wrist, but don't yet make contact with the skin.

2. Very slowly, allow the tiniest amount of the skin of your three fingers to make contact with the tiniest amount, the very surface of the patient's (or your own) skin. You will almost not be touching the skin. Pretend you are barely touching the most delicate butterfly wing. This depth is defined as one bean of pressure.

3. As slowly as possible, add the smallest amount of pressure, almost none at all. Now a bit more, and a bit more. Over a period of about a minute, extremely slowly, move your fingers down into the pulse as slowly as you possibly can.

4. At some point, perhaps about half way through the minute, you'll be aware that you have made contact with the radial artery. Keep going very slowly until you feel you

are in the middle of the artery. This depth is defined as nine beans of pressure.

5. Quite a while after that, you'll feel that if you keep going, you'll stop the flow of blood in the radial artery. Keep going.

6. The flow of blood will stop and very soon after that you'll become aware of the hardness of the bone. Slowly go into the bone. Then keep going until you feel you are compressing the bone a little. This depth is defined as fifteen beans of pressure.

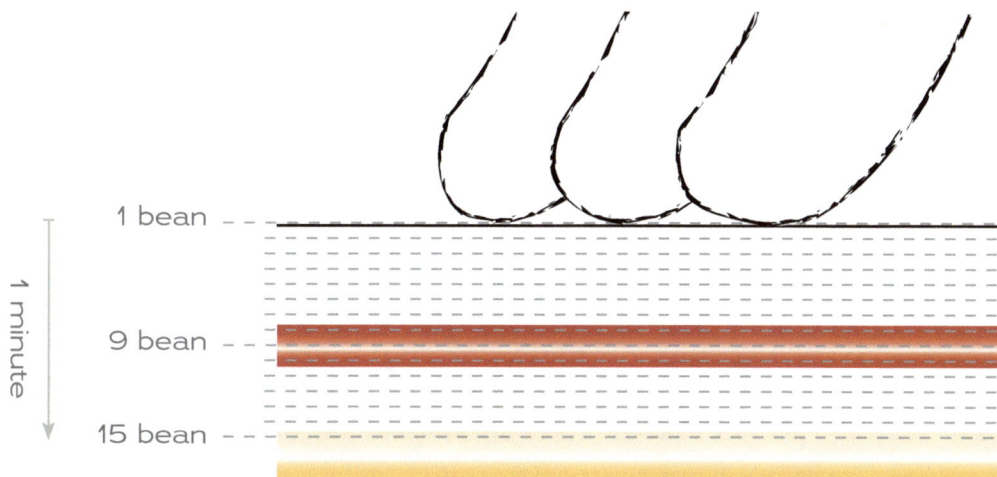

If this exercise is done slowly it's difficult not to be utterly staggered by the magnitude of the distance your finger can travel in the action of moving from the superficial skin through to pressing into the bone. What seems like a small distance becomes a vast arena offering a whole world of information. It's remarkable. In traversing that distance, with practice, it is possible to answer a plethora of diagnostic questions.

From the pulses we are able to discern how well an organ is functioning. As soon as you touch the patient's pulses an interchange begins. Often a pulse feels as though it would like to behave in a different way. By applying focused mental intention the pulses can begin to realign themselves. This doesn't mean we are imposing judgment; rather, it means that the change the pulse is trying to make is being honored and facilitated by the practitioner's intention. Treatment begins before any needles are inserted. If you cannot get a pulse to change by concentrating on it and willing it to change, the condition is in the organ itself, not its associated channel. This section describes the functions of the organs and their detection through probing dynamic pulses. This technique involves varying the depth of an individual finger at an individual position (cun, guan or chi) and noting the response in the pulse at that same position. Whether one chooses probing pulses or directional pulses or both to detect organ function is a matter of personal preference. Some organ functions, however, are best felt using directional pulses. These include the communication between Heart to Kidneys, Kidneys to Heart, Kidneys to Lungs and Lungs to Kidneys.

The Triple Pressure Imperative

All discussion about diagnosis in this manual involves pressure on all three pulse positions. Pulses are not read with pressure applied only to one position because the organ systems are never functioning alone. We always are mindful of the relationships. The default finger depth for the cun and guan positions is the moderate level. The default finger position for the chi position is the deep level. When reading the Liver pulse, for example, the focus is on the guan position while the finger at the cun position is at the moderate level and the finger at the chi position is at the deep level. If the fingers were lifted off the two positions not being considered, the function of the organ being examined would not be clearly shown. The pressure provided by the "idle" fingers simulates the natural internal pressure of the entire physiological system, enabling the pulse taker to get a true picture of the organ in its working context.

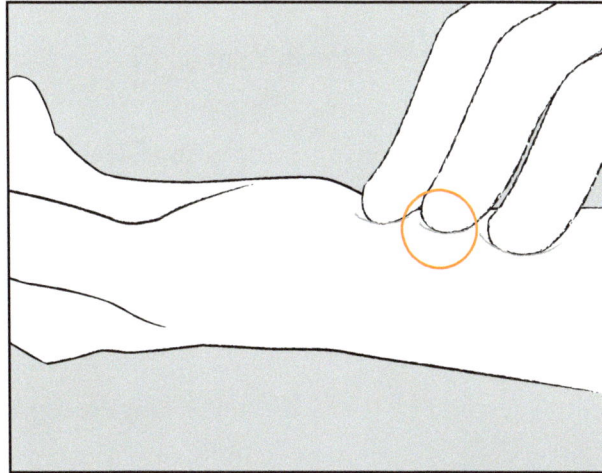

Pressure is maintained in all three positions at all times, even if the practitioner is only focussing on one finger. This simulates the interconnected internal pressures of a working system.

Lung Function and its Presence in the Pulses

The Lung pulse should be strong at the moderate level and should float and disperse, following your finger up to the surface. At the chi position, the Kidneys engender Yang Qi which manifests in the cun position, the Lung pulse. If you push down on the Lung pulse, you should feel it pushing up even more at six beans; it should feel more vibrant. This is part of the floating quality. If it doesn't have a floating quality, then the Spleen needs to be treated to support Wei Qi, because Spleen Yang supports Lung function, or, in another way of seeing, Spleen Yang conducts Kidney Yang Qi up to the Lungs, along with the products of digestion, to be distributed by the Lungs in their role of dispersing. This is what we are looking for in reading the vibrancy of the Lung pulse at six beans, to see whether it has healthy qualities of floating and dispersing.

The Lungs function in order to:
1. Govern Qi
2. Descend Qi
3. Effuse/Diffuse/Disperse Qi
4. Rectify Qi
5. Moisten
6. Move Blood
7. Govern the capacity to let go and forgive or let go and accept.

1. GOVERN QI.

The Lung channel begins at CV-12. A morsel of Yuan Qi stirs the Lungs to fully expand to receive Qi. The Lungs govern Qi in the sense that they receive Qi and let go of Qi.

Pulse Sensation: The moderate level of the pulse should feel strong. This means the connection to the origin of Qi is strong. The Lung pulse should float to confirm that the Lungs can let go of Qi during respiration.

2. DESCEND QI.

After respiration, the Lungs descend Qi to the Kidneys. This descension of Qi enables the opening of the Lower Jiao for conception, menstruation, urination and defecation. The Qi of the Lungs descends to the Kidneys to fan Ming Men, Life Gate at GV-4. This means that the Qi of Heaven permeates us, awakening our destiny within us.

Pulse Sensation: As you press down from the moderate level into the deep level, the Lung pulse should become stronger and fuller at the deep level.

3. EFFUSE/DIFFUSE/DISPERSE QI.

The primary focus of Lung Qi is exhalation. The Lungs are the key organ for letting go of Qi.

Pulse Sensation: The Lung pulse should float. There should be a sense of energy rising. As you release pressure from the pulse at the moderate level, there should be a steady, consistent pressure behind your finger pushing it up to the top of the Wei level. It should float. It is normal for the Lung pulse to be scattered as your finger moves through the Wei level; this is a mark of diffusion.

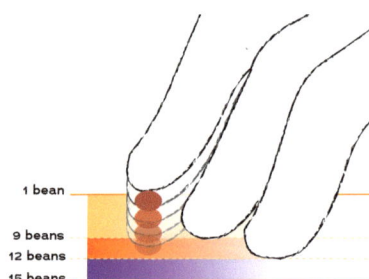

1 bean
9 beans
12 beans
15 beans

4. RECTIFY QI.

This means that a patient is able to discern what is right for him or her, and what is not.

Pulse Sensation: The pulse is strong in the moderate level. It should not be wiry, thin, beady or slippery. This means that the origin of the Lung Channel, CV-12, is strong. There is clarity in the gut generating a knowing of what is right and wrong for the individual. This clarity is unobstructed by dampness.

5. MOISTEN.

The Lungs move Fluids and Blood to moisten.

Pulse Sensation: The pulse is wide at the superficial level indicating that the Lungs are able to move mediumship. The pulse should not be rapid. If the Lungs do not have good width they are not getting Fluids from the Stomach.

6. MOVE BLOOD.

The dispersing function of the Lungs indicates how well they are moving Blood.

Pulse Sensation: This is evident in the degree to which the Lung pulse floats from the moderate to the superficial level.

7. GOVERN THE CAPACITY TO LET GO AND FORGIVE OR LET GO AND ACCEPT.

The Lungs release not only External Pathogenic Factors (EPFs) but control feelings of vulnerability, insecurity, injustice, and the sense of morality.

Pulse Sensation: The pulse should not be wiry or beady. A wiry pulse shows that something cannot be let go. A beady pulse tells us that long-term Phlegm has obstructed the Lungs and their capacity to let go. The Lung pulse should float without feeling slippery. As you release pressure from the pulse at the moderate level, there should be a steady, consistent pressure behind your finger pushing it up to the top of the Wei level. It might scatter as it reaches the Wei level.

PATHOLOGICAL QUALITIES OF THE LUNG PULSE

Generally, the Lungs show pathology if the pulse is not strong at the moderate level, does not disperse, and is beady, tight, wiry or slippery.

Heart Function and its Presence in the Pulses

The Heart pulse should feel full as you raise your finger and relaxed as you push down on it. This means that there is enough Blood for the conduction of experiences and excitement and for the creation of reality. The Heart should have no Yin factors. Yin factors (Damp and Phlegm) hamper its freedom. The Heart should only have Yang pulses. The Heart nourishes the Shen because it is naturally curious and excited. The Heart pulse should be excited, bold and strong, but not rapid.

The Heart functions to:

    1. Govern circulation, the movement of Blood, move Blood to the periphery.

    2. Invigorate Blood.

    3. Open to the tongue.

    4. Share love and joy.

    5. House the Shen.

    6. Open to the eyes.

1. GOVERN CIRCULATION, THE MOVEMENT OF BLOOD, MOVE BLOOD TO THE PERIPHERY.

The optimal circulation of blood allows us to engage in the world and to experience the excitement, joy and interaction the world offers us and that the Heart seeks. The Blood of the Heart seeks human interaction.

Pulse Sensation: The pulse should be strong and full on the moderate level. As the finger is lifted from the deep level, through the moderate level and into the superficial level, the pulse should become stronger and stronger because blood is coming out to the world. The Heart pulse should become full as the finger is on the way up and relaxed as the finger is on the way down.

2. INVIGORATE BLOOD.

Pulse Sensation: The pulse should be strongest at the moderate level, the level of Blood.

3. OPEN TO THE TONGUE.

The Heart opens to the Tongue in order to share joy and express excitement.

Pulse Sensation: The pulse should scatter slightly as it floats to the superficial level from the moderate level.

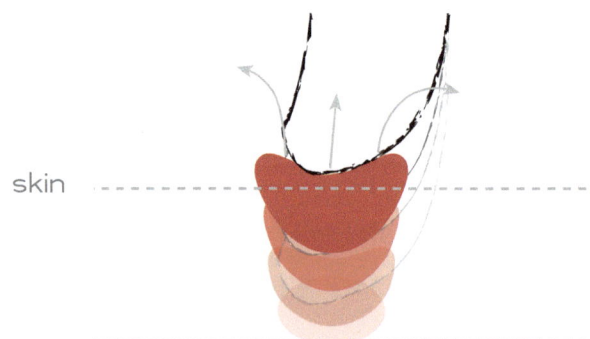

skin

4. SHARE LOVE AND JOY.

This includes the joy experienced in satisfying curiosity and the joy experienced in sharing joy itself. I have found this scattering quality very reliable in determining the patient's level of optimism.

Pulse Sensation: On the superficial level, the Heart pulse scatters slightly, demonstrating the patient's willingness to spread love and joy.

5. HOUSE THE SHEN.

The deep level of the Heart pulse is the location of the retreat of the Shen. Sometimes this pulse will vibrate indicating this retreat as being pathological. But a Shen's retreating nature might also be intrinsic. The deep level illustrates the degree to which the Kidney receives the Yang Qi from the Heart and is able to calm the Shen; the Yang anchors the Shen.

Pulse Sensation: An anchored Shen will show in the deep level of the Heart pulse as relaxed and replete, or even gentle and soft. In this case, the soft pulse is not pathological. An anchored Shen can also show as a Heart pulse that is very slightly tight only at the superficial level. This very superficial tightness is holding the Shen in place. If the pulse at the deep level of the Heart is not relaxed, the patient is unable to calm his or her own Shen, or can't sleep.

6. OPEN TO THE EYES.

To convey excitement and enthusiasm.

Pulse Sensation: The Heart pulse floats. (It follows your finger as you lift it.)

Note that you might find that the Heart pulse has moved up to the superficial level because the patient is delighted to find that you are interested in them. A Heart to Heart conversation, which can be a part of an acupuncture treatment encounter moves the Heart.

PATHOLOGICAL QUALITIES OF THE HEART PULSE

A *wiry Heart pulse* indicates the Heart is constrained. This can be caused by Dampness or Phlegm. Or the patient is knowingly or unknowingly agreeing to a limitation being placed on the amount of joy their Heart is allowed to express.

A *tight pulse* shows obstruction or stagnation in the Heart for similar reasons but at an earlier stage. Sometimes, however, the Heart pulse can be a little tight on the superficial level as the Shen is held in place. This is not pathological.

A *rapid Heart pulse* is showing that there is too much excitement causing Heat. The Heat is in turn preventing the natural nourishment and fulfillment that comes from that very excitement. If the Heart is rapid as it scatters, there is too much stimulation, enough to negatively impact intelligence.

An *urgent Heart pulse* can indicate the presence of an entity.

A *slippery Heart pulse*, especially at the moderate level, means the Spleen is not able to ascend enough Yang to enable the Stomach to adequately ripen and rot; Phlegm in the gut then moves up with the red substance as the red substance is ascended from the Spleen to the Heart. The Phlegm should have been expectorated by the Lungs but the Lungs might have been weak or are currently weak. Resolve Phlegm by strengthening the Spleen, or dissolve it via the Kidneys.

Spleen Function and its Presence in the Pulses

The Spleen pulse naturally is strong with integrity at its borders. It is slightly slippery at the moderate level but not slippery at all in the deep level.

The Spleen functions to:
1. Transform and Transport.
2. Ascend Kidney Yang to the Stomach.
3. Ascend the Pure Yang of the Stomach to the sensory orifices.
4. Ascend Blood to the Heart.
5. Manage blood.
6. Control the Mind.
7. Produce Gu Qi (along with the Stomach).
8. Resolve Dampness and Discharge Dampness.
9. Control the four limbs.
10. Rectify Qi in the Lungs.
11. Support Kidneys in Consolidating Qi.
12. Harmonize with the Stomach.

1. TRANSFORM AND TRANSPORT.

The Spleen maintains fluid metabolism via the process of transformation during the initial process of separation which occurs in the Stomach. The Spleen allows for the extraction of

9

Qi from the fine particles of digestion.

Pulse Sensation: The pulse is strong at the moderate level. The Spleen pulse is naturally very slightly slippery at the moderate level which is the level of the Stomach organ. This is because the Stomach must ripen and rot in order for the Spleen to be able to transform the food. In other words, to be able to cook food (for the Spleen to be able to transform food) one must have the right amount of water (fluids provided by the Stomach). A slippery pulse at the deep level in the Spleen position is pathological, however, because it indicates Dampness in the Spleen itself.

2. ASCEND KIDNEY YANG TO THE STOMACH.

The Spleen provides the ascending movement that brings the Yang of the Kidneys into the digestive tract. This is the Yang required to transform and transport nourishment. Concurrently, the Stomach descends the Qi through the digestive tract.

Pulse Sensation: The descending function of the Stomach is felt as your finger moves from the superficial level to the moderate level. The ascending function of the Spleen is felt as you move down further to the next level, that is, as you press down from the moderate to the deep level the Spleen pulse should become slightly stronger as you press down.

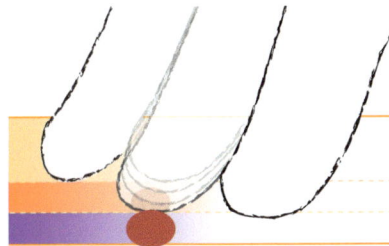

3. ASCEND THE PURE YANG OF THE STOMACH TO THE SENSORY ORIFICES.

The Spleen ascends the pure thin fluids of the Stomach to the sensory orifices so that there is a mediumship to register sight, sound and taste, then to imprint those sensations on the sensory orifices. Without that fluid, life is perceived to be dull.

Pulse Sensation: The ascending function of the Spleen is felt as a slight increase in strength as you move down from the moderate to the deep level.

4. ASCEND BLOOD TO THE HEART.

The Spleen brings the red substance up to the Heart for the finalization of the production of Blood. The Spleen has to store enough red substance at the Stomach in order to transfer it to the Heart for finalization so it can be sent to the Liver to be stored. This blood is delivered to the Liver by the Liver's Jue Yin partner, the Pericardium.

Pulse Sensation: This is a subset of the ascending function of the Spleen. The Spleen pulse should be felt to be slightly stronger as you press from the moderate level to the deep level.

5. MANAGE BLOOD.

The action of holding Blood in its banks is conducted by the Spleen. The Spleen prevents the leakage of Blood.

Pulse Sensation: There is a certain sense of healthy containment in the Spleen pulse. The walls of the vessel in the moderate level feel shored up without being tight. There is good definition in the borders of the Spleen pulse.

6. CONTROL THE MIND.

One of the Spleen's roles is to think about things that are meaningful to the Heart. This is what it really means to bank the Blood. Concentration on these thoughts is in parallel with the literal management or concentration of Blood in the vessels. If thoughts are in keeping with the openness of the Heart, the Spleen has integrity and there will be no hemorrhages or varicosities. The Spleen tempers excessive thinking and resolves that which afflicts the Heart. The Spleen elevates the light that the Heart emanates.

Pulse Sensation: The Spleen pulse has integrity at its sides, feels stable and contained; the walls of the artery feel firm. There is a sense of buoyancy in the moderate level.

7. PRODUCE GU QI (ALONG WITH THE STOMACH).

Gu Qi is a term which means the combination of digestive Qi contained in the chyme and the red substance; in other words, the production of Qi and Blood.

Pulse Sensation: This is felt in the width of the moderate level of the Spleen pulse.

8. RESOLVE DAMPNESS AND DISCHARGE DAMPNESS.

The Spleen resolves Dampness by ensuring there is sufficient Yang being sent upward from the Kidneys to ensure complete digestion.

Pulse Sensation: This function is felt as a slight increase in the strength of the Spleen pulse as the finger presses from the moderate to the deep levels. The Spleen pulse is devoid of slipperiness at the deep level if the Spleen's performance of this function is meeting the demands of the body.

9. CONTROL THE FOUR LIMBS.

The Spleen is responsible for the distribution of Qi to the four limbs, keeping them animated and keeping the hands and feet warm. The four limbs also represent acting out of compassion, walking and moving the arms in order to act out one's life purpose, certain in one's values and beliefs.

Pulse Sensation: Again, the up and out motion of Spleen Qi is felt as a strengthening of the pulse between the moderate and deep levels.

10. RECTIFY QI IN THE LUNGS.

The Spleen rectifies Lung Qi by elevating thoughts to the Lungs to enable the Lungs to let go of pathology (in this case, Phlegm). The Spleen elevates thought to the Lungs to spur them to let go of the phlegm, to forgive, to accept, to let go of afflicting memories.

Pulse Sensation: This is felt as a combination of the ascending vector of the Spleen pulse to the Lungs and the immediate dispersal of Lung Qi, seen as a floating pulse in the Lung position.

11. SUPPORT KIDNEYS IN CONSOLIDATING QI.

The Spleen supports the Kidneys through focus on thoughts that promote self-esteem. The Spleen's elemental partner, the Stomach, then descends this Qi to the Kidneys.

Pulse Sensation: In the right guan position, as you press down from the superficial level to the moderate level, the pulse should become stronger. This shows that the Stomach is descending. At the same time, the Spleen pulse feels as though it has integrity; it ascends confidently. This is demonstrated as the Spleen pulse offers resistance as it is pressed from the moderate to the deep level.

12. HARMONIZE WITH THE STOMACH.

The Spleen ascends Qi, and in so doing enables its elemental partner the Stomach to descend Qi.

Pulse Sensation: Descension of the Stomach is demonstrated as your finger goes from superficial to moderate and experiences a strengthening of the pulse. The ascension of the Spleen is shown as a resistance against the finger that emerges as the finger moves from the moderate level to deep level. If these two sensations match, the Spleen and the Stomach are harmonized.

Liver Function and its Presence in the Pulses

The Liver pulse is naturally slightly tight at the moderate level, especially between six and nine beans. Sometimes it is tighter in women because its principal function is to gather and store Blood. It should not be wiry, as that would indicate stagnation. There is a natural softness at the deep level. The pulse does not become thinner as it is pressed more deeply, especially when pressed beyond 12 beans. The Liver pulse maintains integrity throughout the entire depth of the pulse until you reach beyond 12 beans when it starts to disintegrate as its blood is broken down to nourish Jing-Essence. It shows ascension in moving up with your finger when you raise it and descension by pressing up against your finger as you move your finger downward. The Liver pulse should not scatter, as that indicates Wind in the Liver.

The Liver functions to:
1. Regulate Qi.
2. Engender Heart Qi.
3. Engender Heart Blood.
4. Course or Spread the Qi.
5. Regulate the smooth flow of Qi.
6. Store Blood.
7. Discharge Dampness, especially Damp Heat.
8. Bring Blood to the Sinews.
9. Bring Blood to the Brain.
10. Open to the Eyes.
11. Plan.
12. House the Hun (the collective conscious) and store memories or images of the past, present and future.
13. Nourish the Kidneys.
14. Nourish the structure, hair and nails.
15. Send Blood to the Kidneys to foster self-worth.
16. Bring Blood to the Lower Jiao for Fertility and Creativity.

1. REGULATE QI.

Pulse Sensation: The vectors of ascension and descension are felt equally; as you lift your finger, the pulse follows the finger up and as you apply more pressure the pulse continues to have integrity, although it will soften in the deep level. This is normal.

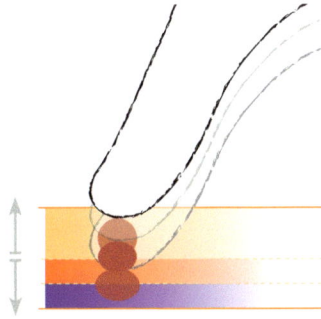

2. ENGENDER HEART QI.

Liver Blood not only becomes Jing-Essence or Kidney Yin, it also becomes Heart Qi. The Liver gives the Heart the resources it needs to find things interesting, to find life interesting. The Heart and the Liver both go to the eyes. The eyes reveal new things to the Heart and the Liver provides the resources to create achievements in relation to what is seen. Heart Qi draws upon Liver Blood, using the Liver's resources to create action and bring about the realization of one's destiny or life's purpose.

Pulse Sensation: As you lift your finger slowly from the moderate level, the pulse energetically follows you.

3. ENGENDER HEART BLOOD.

Pulse Sensation: As you lift your finger within the moderate level, the pulse feels wide and plentiful.

4. COURSE OR SPREAD THE QI.

The Liver is responsible for the spreading of Qi through both Yin and Yang Sinews, which in turn control all the smooth muscle and the exterior.

Pulse Sensation: The Liver is slightly tight, but not wiry, and is able to follow your finger up and remain strong as you push your finger back down into the pulse.

5. REGULATE THE SMOOTH FLOW OF QI.

The Liver controls the diaphragm, which must be relaxed in order to maintain the smooth flow of Qi. A stagnated Liver can oppress the diaphragm.

Pulse Sensation: The Liver pulse might feel slightly tight but the top of the pulse comes up into your finger. It is not circumferentially tight.

6. STORE BLOOD.

The Liver stores blood. Most of one's Blood is returned to the Liver with every heart beat during sleep.

Pulse Sensation: The Liver is shown to be storing Blood when the Liver pulse is slightly tight, or tight at between six and nine beans of pressure. To store Blood there must be Qi at the Liver position; it cannot be weak.

7. DISCHARGE DAMPNESS, ESPECIALLY DAMP HEAT.

The Liver usually discharges Dampness by generating diarrhea. This is its detoxifying method. The Gallbladder is used to hasten this discharge and move the stagnation.

Pulse Sensation: The Liver shows it is able to discharge Dampness when the pulse is felt to maintain its integrity in the moderate level and soften when pressed to the deep level. This is normal.

8. BRING BLOOD TO THE SINEWS.

Pulse Sensation: The pulse follows your finger upward from the moderate level to within the upper level of the pulse.

9. BRING BLOOD TO THE BRAIN.

Liver Blood nourishes the brain via the internal branch that connects the Liver to the brain and terminates at GV-20.

Pulse Sensation: The pulse follows your finger as you move from the moderate level up to three beans of pressure. The Liver is ascending Blood to the brain.

10. OPEN TO THE EYES.

via the first branch of the Liver Primary Channel.

Pulse Sensation: The pulse follows your finger as you move from the moderate level up to three beans of pressure.

11. PLAN.

The Liver stores Blood which in turn stores memory. This enables the Liver to plan. (The Liver plans, planning is Yin; the Gallbladder is the decision maker, deciding is Yang.)

Pulse Sensation: The Liver pulse is slightly tight. It is not wiry; a stagnated Liver cannot be flexible enough to plan.

12. HOUSE THE HUN.

(the collective conscious) and store memories or images of the past, present and future.

Pulse Sensation: The pulse is slightly tight between nine and six beans of pressure. The sides of the pulse have integrity.

13. NOURISH THE KIDNEYS.

Blood from the Liver nourishes the Kidneys. This is one of the few ways postnatal Qi nourishes Jing-Essence.

Pulse Sensation: There must be Qi available in order to store Blood. A weak Liver pulse indicates that there is insufficient Qi to store Blood and so Liver Blood cannot be nourishing the Kidneys. If the Liver pulse is weak on the deep level, the Liver is not supporting the Essence and the structure. At 12 beans there should be softness in the pulse. Beyond that the pulse should almost feel as though it is disintegrating as Blood breaks apart to nourish the Essence. The Liver softens the Blood so that it can become Jing.

Note: (The softness described above should not be confused with weakness. The soft pulse that is weak is the one that is felt just beneath a floating pulse, indicating that Wei Qi is not being supported by Fluids.)

14. NOURISH THE STRUCTURE, HAIR AND NAILS.

Pulse Sensation: At 12 beans of pressure the pulse is not at all weak. If at this deep level it is weak, frail, empty or minute, the Liver is not supporting the structure, the hair or the nails. The weakness indicates the Liver has inadequate Qi which is required to store Blood and to move that Blood down to the Kidneys to support Jing-Essence.

15. SEND BLOOD TO THE KIDNEYS TO FOSTER SELF-WORTH.

Self-esteem is a function of Jing-Essence as it is stored in the Kidneys. Jing is replenished through postnatal Qi as Liver Blood nourishes Jing.

Pulse Sensation: At 12 beans there should be softness in the pulse and just beyond that the pulse should almost feel as though it is disintegrating as Blood breaks apart to nourish Jing-Essence. The Liver softens the Blood so that it can become Jing.

16. BRING BLOOD TO THE LOWER JIAO FOR FERTILITY AND CREATIVITY.

A shortage of Liver Blood moving to the genitalia to create Kidney Yin results in impotence, infertility and a lack of creativity.

Pulse Sensation: At 12 beans there should be a soft quality. (Soft does not mean weak.) At 12 beans you should begin to feel a meshing of the Blood and Jing levels. This is the juncture at which the Blood becomes Jing-Essence. If there's a melding here and a concurrent softening, the Blood is becoming denser, becoming Yin. The pulse should break apart when pressing deeper than 12 beans.

Pathological Qualities of the Liver Pulse

A wiry pulse indicates stagnation of Liver Qi. The Liver is not storing Blood. Stagnation of the Liver also prevents the smooth flow of Qi and many other Liver functions. A wiry pulse can result from long term tightness from Cold. The impact of Cold on the Liver pulse can be very strong but it is not to be mistaken for strength; it is merely extreme tightness and the fight that has ensued to break up that Cold and push it out to the exterior. Extreme tightness can indicate late Shao Yin or Jue Yin pathology. Initially the pulse could be slow also, but in the long term it can be wiry. Wiry pulses show that Liver Blood cannot nourish the Heart or the Kidneys. Ultimately this can lead to a lack of interest in learning and in life as the Heart is not nourished. This can affect the patient's sense of self-worth and lead to shyness, timidity and apprehension, doubt and uncertainty. Moxa LR-12 to break up Cold in the Liver. Note that wiry should not be confused with tight. A wiry pulse is circumferentially tight; a tight pulse is tight at the sides.

A *thin* Liver pulse indicates the Liver is not storing enough Blood to be able to nourish the Heart and Kidneys.

A *rapid* Liver pulse. The Liver pulse should not be rapid. Heat would then be free to rise to the Heart.

A *slow* Liver pulse. The Liver pulse should not be slow. This would show that the Liver is stagnated and unable to effectively move Blood up or down.

A *scattered* Liver pulse indicates that internal Wind is present. Wind needs to be coursed or subdued. (If the Hun is not stable, calm the Shen with GB-9 and GB-13, even technique.)

A *floating* Liver pulse indicates that Yang is floating. Yang needs to be subdued or anchored.

A Liver pulse that is full in the superficial level indicates Yang is not anchored.

A *weak* Liver pulse shows that the Liver is not able to store Blood.

A *slippery Liver pulse* indicates an imbalance between the Liver and the Spleen. Treat the Spleen since the Spleen is not controlling Damp.

A *choppy Liver pulse* indicates the Liver is attempting to astringe (tighten its Qi around) Blood but there is insufficient Blood to store. This feels like an accordion under your finger as it dilates and tightens, dilates and tightens.

Kidney Function and its Presence in the Pulses

The Kidney pulses are felt at the deep level where they naturally are slightly tight, as their principal function is to conserve Jing-Essence. They should feel strong and full.

When pressure is released from the deep level, the pulse should follow your finger to the cusp of the moderate level. The Kidney pulse should feel strong there as well.

A Kidney pulse felt at the superficial level is pathological. To a lesser degree a Kidney pulse felt at the moderate level is also pathological.

The Kidney Yin pulse, felt on the left side, is called the stone pulse; it is naturally tight, slow and heavy as it seeks to conserve Jing-Essence. The slowness is not to be confused with Cold. Cold is simply the nature of Jing, and is supposed to be conserved and used sparingly.

The Kidney Yang pulse which is on the right should be faster than its Yin partner. Kidney Yang is the foundation of warmth, movement and enthusiasm for life. It provides the movement needed to disseminate Jing-Essence to the Bladder Shu points, maintaining the minute-to-minute functioning of the organs. A rapid Kidney Yang pulse at the deep level might not be pathological but might indicate great enthusiasm for life. The Kidney Yang pulse should simply be strong.

The Kidney Yang pulse should not be any more than slightly tight, if it is tight at all. If it is tight it may be acting to prevent leakage.

The Kidney pulse can be slightly soft when the patient is in deep contemplation or in a state of deep relaxation.

The Kidneys Function to:
   1. Control Reproduction.
   2. Control Growth, Decay and Decline.

3. House the Zhi-Will.

4. Consolidate and Secure the Essence.

5. Maintain the bones, structure, shape and form.

6. Regulate the Waterways.

7. Receive Qi.

8. Control the lower orifices.

9. Disseminate Yang Qi.

1. CONTROL REPRODUCTION.

The Kidneys secure the Essence, ensuring the storage of the resources necessary for procreation.

Pulse Sensation: The Kidney Yin pulse (left) is slightly tight.

2. CONTROL GROWTH, DECAY AND DECLINE.

The Kidneys secure the Jing-Essence so that Jing is not wasted, its decline not hastened. This optimizes the availability of Jing for the carrying out of growth bound in one's destiny.

Pulse Sensation: The Kidney Yin pulse (left) is slightly tight.

3. HOUSE THE ZHI-WILL.

The Zhi-Will is what encourages us to be who we truly are, rather than what society might dictate. The role of the Zhi is to navigate the true path of destiny and to ensure that we are true to ourselves.

Pulse Sensation: As you press more into the deep level the Kidney pulse should become stronger.

4. CONSOLIDATE AND SECURE THE ESSENCE.

The security of the Jing-Essence is dependent on one's endorsement of oneself. The Jing is secure if one can squarely say to oneself that they appreciate themselves, that they have a real love of the self. It is impossible to be true to oneself, to be authentic, if there is not love of the self. If there is self-loathing, or if there is the underlying feeling of shame about who one is, the Jing is consumed. Fire runs rampant as it is unbalanced and burning the Jing.

Pulse Sensation: As you press deeper into the deep level the Kidney pulse should become stronger. It should not become stronger as you raise your finger to the moderate level. That would indicate there is insufficient Qi to hold or to move the Yin down. This applies to the Yang and the Yin Kidney pulses.

5. MAINTAIN THE BONES, STRUCTURE, SHAPE AND FORM.

The Kidneys govern the way Jing-Essence is meted out to become our structure.

Pulse Sensation: As you press deeper into the deep level the Kidney pulse should become stronger.

6. REGULATE THE WATERWAYS.

The Kidneys determine how rapidly water will flow and change from a liquid state to a more solid state as it become Jing-Essence. (This movement is also regulated by the Yang Qi of Triple Heater and the Bladder Channel.) Triple Heater regulates the temperature of water, lowering it to allow water to become Jing and raising it to enable it to become Qi. During this process, turbid water must be moved so that it does not decay; Kidney Yang provides the movement for this process.

Pulse Sensation: The right Kidney pulse is strong and energetic in the deep level. It has good width.

7. RECEIVE QI.

The Kidneys are responsible for the reception of Qi. In the Kidney position, the reception of Stomach Qi and Lung Qi is felt.

Pulse Sensation: You might feel something in the moderate level of the Kidney pulse as you are diagnosing the reception of Qi. This is because the moderate level is the level of postnatal Qi and your focus is on the movement of Qi from that level down to the Kidneys. But during the process of moving your finger down from the moderate level to the deep level of the Kidney pulse, that is, from nine beans down to 15 beans of pressure, the pulse should become strong and fuller. This shows that the contract of life is accepted and the Qi of Heaven and of Humanity is accepted. Note that the emergence of the fullness and strength is not evident at 15 beans of pressure, but evident during the journey your finger makes from nine beans to 15 beans.

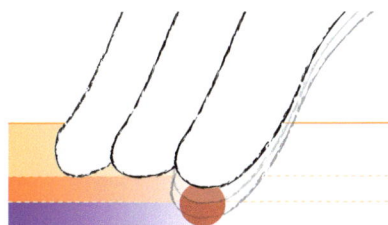

If the Lungs and Stomach are not descending it means the Lungs and Stomach are not nourishing Kidney Qi. The Lungs and the Stomach are the postnatal receptors and they must both descend to support Kidney Qi. It is important to determine which of the two organs is not descending and then to treat that organ's function.

8. CONTROL THE LOWER ORIFICES.
The Kidneys control the urethra and anus.

Pulse Sensation: The Kidney Yang pulse (right) feels solid and anchored in the deep position. Its borders are well-defined.

9. DISSEMINATE YANG QI.
Kidney Yang is the foundation of the temperament. Ming Men supports the carrying out of a life's mandate. The Kidneys provide the Yang Qi to the Triple Heater to enable the dissemination of Jing-Essence to the Bladder Shu points which in turn transport that Jing to the organs for the expression of life.

Pulse Sensation: The pulse is anchored in the deep level and is not floating and scattered. As you release pressure from the deep to the bottom of the moderate level the pulse follows you but remains strong.

Pathological Qualities of the Kidney Pulse
A weak Kidney pulse shows the Kidney is unable to consolidate Jing-Essence.

A rapid left Kidney (Yin) pulse shows that Jing-Essence is being rapidly combusted.

A wiry Kidney pulse shows there is stagnation of the Jing-Essence; Jing is not being disseminated.

A scattered Kidney Yang pulse indicates escaping Yang.

A floating Kidney pulse in either position also means Yang is escaping.

A slow, wiry pulse in the Kidney Yang pulse can indicate Cold or stagnation.

A slow Kidney Yang pulse shows Cold or stagnation of Yang Qi. The Kidney Yang pulse should not have a quality that hampers movement.

A tight Kidney Yang pulse indicates that a Yin factor is hampering the movement of Yang.

A floating, tight Kidney pulse means the body is trying to stem leakage of Jing-Essence or Yin. As it escapes, Zong-Ancestral-Gathering Qi tries to anchor the Qi back down, making the pulse floating and tight.

21

Yang-Fu Organ Function in the Pulses

The Fu organs are seen as the Yang aspect, or extensions of the Zang organs, and are used to augment the Yang functions of the Zang organs. The Fu organs provide movement for the Zang organs and have the capacity to bring pathology out of latency, that is, suppressed pathology originating in trauma and the suppression of the personality. For example, Large Intestine points bring out pathology of the Lungs' metal quality or even personality traits pertaining to the Lungs. The Small Intestine and Triple Heater move pathology in the Heart and Pericardium and bring out fire qualities in the personality. The Heart spreads its Qi but is loathe to do so in the presence of Yin factors such as Damp and Cold, but the Small Intestine can dissipate Cold, Wind, Damp and Clear Heat; it deals with climatic factors.

Reading the Fu Organs

To Read the Fu Organs:

1. Press all three fingers to the moderate level.
2. Focus on one pulse position while maintaining pressure in the moderate level on the other two positions.
3. Decide whether the sensation you are feeling pertains to the Yang-Fu organ or the Yin-Zang organ. This is done by considering the major functions of the Zang and the Fu organs and locating the corresponding quality or lack thereof in the pulse. Most of the Fu organs do not have many major roles and so this is not nearly as complex as the reading of the Zang organs.

Note: The function of the Fu organs is to move, to discharge, to dissipate (break up) and to release and drain pathologies of their Zang partner. They perform the Yang functions of the pulse position. Therefore rapid pulses in the deep level are pertaining to the Fu organ of that position. This is telling us that the Fu organ is trying to move the pathology contained in the Zang organ of that position.

4. If the quality that pertains to the Fu organs which is found at the moderate level seems to be mirrored in the superficial level or if it seems to extend into the superficial level as a continuous sensation, we can say that we are feeling the Fu organ. Also if a quality pertaining to the Fu organ is found on the deep level and is extending up to the superficial level, we can say the Fu organ is being felt and also that it is very active.

For example, the Large Intestine dissipates Wind and clears Heat. LU-10 can clear Heat, but the Large Intestine can clear Heat more efficiently because the Yang Channels have a greater capacity for moving things out. (Yin has, by contrast of course, a greater capacity to store.) A rapid pulse felt in the deep or moderate level of the Lung pulse that extends up to the superficial level is showing you that the Heat contained in the Lung organ at the deep level is being moved out to the exterior via the Large Intestine.

The Bladder organ can be felt in right at the cusp of the Ying and Yuan levels, at about 12 beans of pressure.

Ascension of the Stomach (Advanced)

This ascension is discernible as a resistance in the pulse between 9 and 12 beans of pressure in the right guan position. The Stomach's main function is to descend Qi. It moves food and Gu Qi down the digestive tract and connects with its Yang Ming partner the Large Intestine. But there is also an ascending component to the Stomach, as another of its major functions is the provision of Jin-Thin Fluids which are ascended via Chong Mai from ST-42 to the sensory orifices. It is the Stomach that provides the mediumship that allows us to have a "lens" to perceive the world. This includes the fluids for perception in the sinuses, the nasal cavity, the taste buds and the aural cavities. If this fluid is not ascended effectively everything looks lackluster or polluted; nothing seems exciting. This elevation goes through the Heart since Chong is involved and so the Heart is also elevated. This is how we are able to perceive beauty. The capacity of the Heart to be excited or enthusiastic about life depends on the capacity of the Stomach to ascend its Pure Yang (pure Jin-Thin fluids).

Earlier we saw that the general descension of Stomach Qi is felt as a strengthening of the pulse as you push from the superficial to the moderate level. We also saw that the ascension of the Spleen is felt as a resistance as you continue pressing through the moderate level and into the deep level. In very advanced pulse taking, the ascending function of the Stomach is felt in the first part of that continued pressing, that is, the first part of the resistance which would be between 9 and 12 beans of pressure. Beyond (deeper than) 12 beans you are feeling purely the ascending function of the Spleen.

FREQUENTLY ASKED QUESTION

If the Yin organs are felt at the deep level of the pulse, how can it be that we are detecting Yang organ function at the deep level?

The Yang organs function as extensions of the Yin organs to move pathology away from the Yin organs. If a rapid quality is felt at the deep level and that quality extends upward in the pulse to the moderate or superficial level, it is telling us that the Yang organ is functioning in its capacity to clear pathology from that Yin organ.

Part 2

Directional Pulses and Organ Communication

Historical Roots of Directional Pulses

Directional pulses are a feature of Chapter 11, Scroll 5 of Wang Shu He's second century CE text, the *Mai Jing* (The Pulse Classic). In this book appear the practices of the most prominent practitioners in the Han Dynasty: Hua To and Zhang Zhong Jing (who, incidentally, were competitors) and Bian Que. By the time of the Song Dynasty, directional pulses had disappeared and only static pulses remained. This is partly because the complement channels—the Sinew, Luo, Divergent and Eight Extraordinary Channels—had gone into disuse by that time. Hence, Li Shi Zhen's famous pulse book describes only static pulses, 27 in all.

The practice of directional pulses was not lost, however, from the time of the *Mai Jing*. These teachings, no doubt in somewhat varying forms, were preserved in oral lineages often protected by rules of discipleship. The way in which these pulses were practiced has been in the hands of a rare few individuals since the Song Dynasty, and so this chapter comprises perhaps the most treasured information I am sharing in this volume. It is certainly the information I am most excited about and find invaluable every hour in my clinic. I hope that it will profoundly expand your pulse inquiries.

STATIC AND DIRECTIONAL PULSES

Static pulse taking is very widely used and can provide essential information. Specifically, static pulses tell us the status and quantities of Qi and mediumship. They are single, focused inquiries and are read without moving the finger. The pulse is read at any of the positions and any of the three general depths. Observations about its quality and rate are made, but no inquiry is made about the behavior of that pulse in response to the movement of the practitioner's finger.

Directional pulses, by contrast, involve the practitioner's generation of hydraulic actions in the radial artery. These movements involve one, two or three fingers, and resemble a pumping action. Both static and directional pulses are important, but directional pulses readily provide information regarding communication between organs. Static pulses, read without moving the finger, tell us the status and quantities of Qi and mediumship. If we only have information from static pulses, we need to rely on other diagnostics or intuition because static pulses do not tell us where the pathology is coming from or where it is going. It is likely that we can't even be sure where the pathology is. This is because compromised functioning of a channel or an organ can create effects in another channel or organ. In static pulse taking, when the finger depresses a pulse that pulse position is isolated; it is not communicating with its neighboring organ. Therefore one is not able to see the dynamic exchange between two or more pulses—the dynamic conversation between organs. In static pulses we are also unable to see the dynamic movements between the various depths of the pulse, since each depth is inquired about separately, if at all.

THE IMPORTANCE OF DIRECTIONAL PULSES

Directional pulses are derived from the basic concept that function creates form. In Chinese medicine perhaps the clearest manifestation of this idea occurs in the musculoskeletal system; the way in which we use our body causes it to form in a certain way. For example, the skeletal structure of an obese person has to shift and change to accommodate a weight distribution for which it was not built. A heavy backpack worn habitually only on one shoulder can cause that shoulder to shift and become lower than the other; the function required of the shoulder has affected the actual structure of the shoulder. Similarly, the way in which an organ is performing creates the shape of the pulse. Movements of the finger enable us to read the shape of the pulse in order to see the function (the action) that created the (static) form.

Directional pulses tell us whether there is a problem with the actual organ or whether the pathology is resulting from a failure of communication between organs. If a "directional" action of the finger in one position fails to produce a response in another position, we can deduce that the pathology is in the organ itself, not the channel. If you cannot generate communication between two given pulses using the actions of your fingers, or if you can't create communication in the pulses using spoken dialogue with the patient, there exists an actual visceral organ problem. For example, if the pulse is rapid at a deep level and you can't change it with palpation of the pulses or dialogue with the patient as you are taking the pulses, it's likely there is Heat in the organ itself.

Directional pulses are invaluable in determining the class of channel to be treated and then the exact channel within that class. They also tell us which medium needs to be tended in order for a treatment to be successful. In directional pulses, changes within the position and changes between positions are noted. If the guan position is released, perhaps the cun changes, perhaps the chi changes. These changes reflect the quality of communication between the organs. The early masters were particularly interested in these observations.

Directional pulses reveal the location of excesses and deficiencies. Wherever there is an excess there will be a deficiency and vice versa. We can see whether a wiry or a tight pulse is present due to a pathogenic factor (cold) or whether the tightness is a healthy reaction of the body as it rectifies the lack of something, such as the deficiency of a humor. This kind of information is crucially important since the correct treatments for either possibility are virtually polar opposites of each other. In the first case we would be scattering cold, but in the second case we would be aggressively nourishing the deficient medium—two very different treatments for different causes of a tight or wiry pulse. To unblock an accumulation (tightness) if it is present due to a deficiency would result in the loss of more mediumship and a worsening of the condition. The information gleaned in these pulses can be the difference between a treatment that is a complete success and one that is way off the mark.

Organ Function in Directional Pulses

THE BREADTH OF INQUIRY

The following list describes the inquiries made in the examination of Directional Pulses.

1. Are the Lungs capable of Dispersing?
2. Does Spleen Qi ascend to the Lungs?
3. Is Triple Heater expressing something from the Jing?
4. Is Kidney Yang escaping?
5. Does Stomach Qi descend to the intestines?
6. Does Lung Qi descend to the Kidneys to nourish postnatal Qi?
7. Does Lung Yin descend to the Kidneys to nourish Kidney Yin?
8. Does Kidney Yang finance Wei Qi to enable the Lungs to perform their dispersing function?
9. Does Heart Qi disperse?
10. Do Liver Qi and Liver Blood ascend to engender Heart Qi and Heart Blood?
11. Does Liver Blood Descend to the Kidneys to nourish Kidney Yin?
12. Does the Heart communicate to the Kidneys?
13. Do the Kidneys communicate to the Heart?

THE IMPORTANCE OF THE ABOVE FINDINGS:

1. *The Lungs disperse Qi.*
   This function enables the Lungs to expel External Pathogenic Factors (EPFs). It is a measure of the readiness and effectiveness of the immune system.

2. *Spleen Qi finances Lung Qi by ascending its Qi to the Lungs.*
   The Spleen ascends its Qi to support Lung Qi. Lung Qi is determined by the adequacy of the connection between the Middle Jiao and the Lungs.

3. *Triple Heater moves pathology out of the Jing.*
   Triple Heater moves pathology from the Yuan level out to the Wei level for elimination.

4. *Stomach Qi descends to the intestines.*
   The downward motion of intestinal function comes from the Stomach.

5. *Lung Qi descends to the Kidneys.*
   The Lungs descend Qi with the assistance of Yin from the Heart. This is the postnatal origin of Kidney Qi and Kidney Yin.

6. *Lung Yin descends to the Kidneys.*
   The Lungs descend Yin to the Kidneys to nourish Yin.

7. *The Lungs gather reinforcements of Yang Qi from the Kidneys.*
   The Kidneys grasp Lung Qi. Yang Qi is engendered at the chi position of the right hand and manifests at the Cun position of the right hand. That is to say that the Kidneys support Lung Qi. If Wei Qi (which is controlled by the Lungs) is not able to deal with a pathogenic factor, Wei Qi then retreats to the chest where the Lungs (and Zhong Qi) reorientate to the bowels to cause urination and defecation of the pathogen. During this process, the Lungs descend to the Kidneys either to recycle Wei Qi (returning it to Kidney Yang which is on the right side) or the Lungs descend to the Kidneys to gather more Wei Qi, to reinforce Lung Qi. (Interestingly this language originates from the end of the Warring States period and the Western Jin period when reinforcements were needed in warfare.) The Lungs, like an emissary, communicate with the Kidneys to obtain reinforcements and then ascend with those reinforcements in hand. We need to make sure the Lungs are able to access the Yang Qi. This is seen at the deep level of the chi position.

8. *The Heart disperses Qi.*
   The Heart's main function is to shine its great light outward.

9. *Liver Qi and Liver Blood ascend to engender Heart Qi and Heart Blood.*

Heart Blood and Qi are derived from Liver Blood.

10. *Liver Blood descends to the Kidneys to nourish Kidney Yin.*

Liver Blood is a postnatal origin of Kidney Yin.

11. *The Heart communicates to the Kidneys.*

The Heart shines its light to the Kidneys, bringing illumination and self-reflection to the unknown.

12. *The Kidneys communicate to the Heart.*

The Kidneys reveal the curriculum of life to the Heart which in turn meets the inherent challenges with its beam of shining light.

DIRECTIONAL PULSE TAKING METHOD

At first, this chapter will seem complicated. It's not, really. I've included as many diagrams as possible. Fortunately, once you grasp the movement of Spleen Qi to the Lungs you have the main building block for the whole system. The rest of the process is merely duplicating the same action in different positions. After a short while it becomes easy to perform the actions. I'm sure you will find the result quite remarkable and its addition to your practice invaluable.

POSITIONING THE FINGERS FOR DIRECTIONAL PULSE TAKING

Pulse Neutral Position

The starting position for directional pulse taking is a position I call Pulse Neutral. The fingers in the cun and guan positions sit at 9 beans of pressure (squarely in the moderate level of the pulse) and the finger at the chi position is at 12 beans of pressure (at the interface of Ying and Yuan Qi).

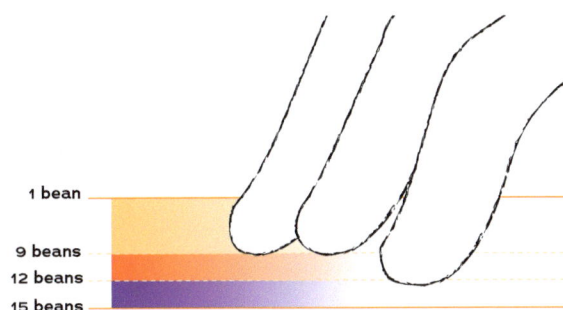

1 bean
9 beans
12 beans
15 beans

The Tilt and Release Actions

Directional pulses measure vectors, that is, the direction in which mediumship and Qi are moving. Directional pulses involve two types of action: the tilt and the release.

The Tilt Action and the Pop

The tilt action is a compound movement made by two fingers. At the same time that one finger is moving down (toward the bone) another finger is moving up (away from the bone). The resulting hydraulic action in the artery causes an accent on the pulse at the finger being lifted. I call this the "pop". The pop is a surge of energy. The pop affects one single beat of the pulse.

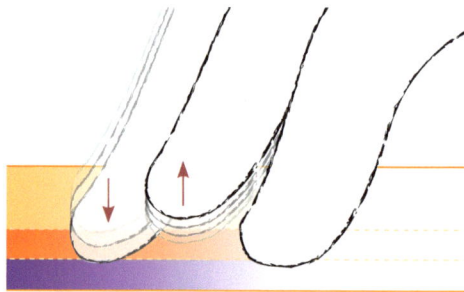

The finger action in the tilt is extremely tiny. Often, when I teach this technique, students say at first that they cannot see or feel the action of my fingers on their wrist. After a few minutes, their attention is honed and they can feel it. It's just a matter of focus, of finely tuned attention.

To practice the action away from the pulse, however, use gross actions, just to get orientated. The resting position for the tilt action is 9 beans in the cun and guan, and 12 beans in the chi position.

The range of motion in the tilt is about three beans in either direction. The cun and guan fingers are at times going to move up toward 6 beans of pressure or down toward 12 beans of pressure.

The chi finger will at times move down toward 15 beans and sometimes up toward 9 beans of pressure.

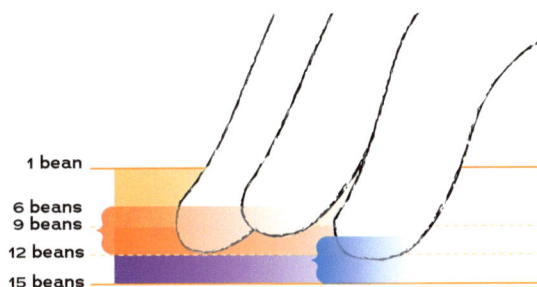

With practice, these actions become smaller and smaller and the readings can be done with movements of three beans or fewer, up or down.

The Release Action

The release action tests for floating pulses. To practice it, go to 12 beans at the right cun position. Very, very slowly release your pressure. Allow the journey from nine beans to one bean to take about 30 seconds. Some pulses reveal pathology when they float. Others reveal pathology when they do not float. When focusing on a pulse that should float, I write down the degree to which a pulse is in fact floating, based on how far it comes up. For example, if the Lung pulse floats from nine beans to one bean, I'll write "100%" on the chart. If it floats up to six beans and then is lost under the fingers, I'll write "30%" on the chart.

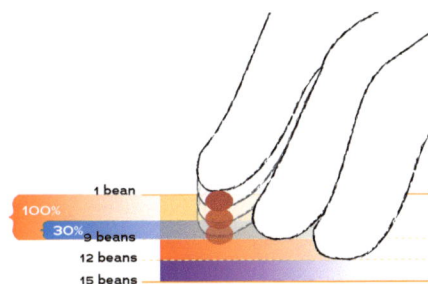

THE SEQUENCE OF DIRECTIONAL PULSES

Note: Directional pulses are just one part of a full pulse diagnosis. See chapter 6 for fully comprehensive step by step protocols.

1. Assume pulse neutral position.

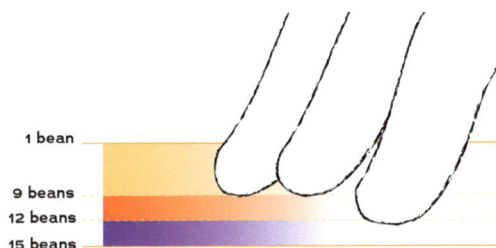

30

2. Release: Are the Lungs capable of Dispersing their Qi to maintain the distribution of Wei Qi? As slowly as possible release pressure from the Lung pulse and allow your finger to follow the pulse upward toward the skin. The pulse should follow your finger all the way up to skin level—to one bean—and may scatter at that point.

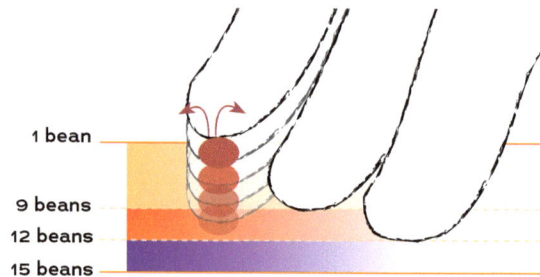

a. If the Lung pulse does follow your finger all the way to the surface, we can say that the Lungs are fully dispersing Qi.

b. If the Lung pulse does not follow your finger all the way to the surface, we can say that the Lungs are not fully dispersing Qi. If you are going very slowly and yet lose the pulse under your finger at, for example, the half way mark, you could say the Lungs are dispersing to about 50% of capacity.

3. Tilt: Does Spleen Qi ascend to the Lungs, to finance Lung Qi? Simultaneously press both the Spleen and Kidney pulses down the tiniest amount and at the same time release the tiniest amount of pressure from the Lung pulse. The Lung pulse should give one pop during the next beat.

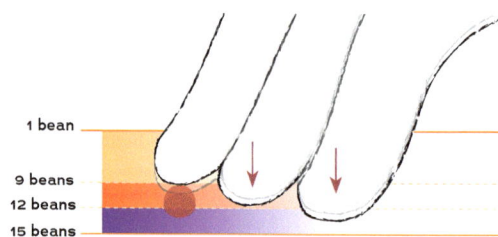

a. If the Lung pulse does pop, we can say that Spleen Qi does ascend to the Lungs.

b. If the Lung pulse does not pop, we can say that Spleen Qi does not ascend to the Lungs.

4. Release: Is Triple Heater expressing something from the Jing? Is Kidney Yang escaping? As slowly as possible, release pressure from the Kidney Yang pulse (right chi) and

allow your finger to follow the pulse upward toward the skin. The pulse should stop following the finger while still within the Yuan level. If it stays in contact with your finger as you lift it, keep going and note the point at which it stops following the finger.

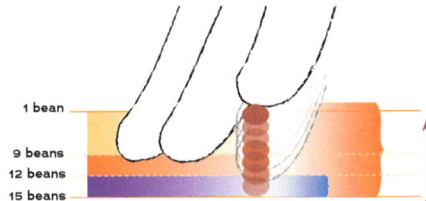

a. If the pulse is lost within the moderate level, we can say there is imbalance in the Pericardium and its facilitation of the communication of Heart and Kidneys.

b. If the pulse comes up to the Wei level, we can say that Kidney Yang is escaping.

c. If the pulse comes up to the top of the Wei level and is very rapid, we can say that the Triple Heater mechanism is engaged in trying to eradicate pathology from the Yuan level.

5. Tilt: Does Stomach Qi descend to the intestines? From the neutral position, press the Spleen pulse down the tiniest amount and at the same time, release the tiniest amount of pressure from the Kidney pulse. The Kidney pulse should give one pop during the next beat.

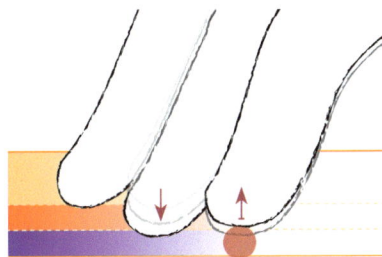

a. If the Kidney pulse does pop we can say that Stomach Qi does descend.

b. If the Kidney pulse does not pop, we can say that the Stomach is not descending or not descending optimally.

c. If the Stomach is not descending and the vector from Spleen to Lungs seems overly pronounced, the Stomach might be ascending; you may be finding rebellious Stomach Qi. To find out if this is the case, raise your cun and guan fingers a few beans and check the guan position to cun position vector at a more superficial level. If it still pronounced, there is rebellious Qi of the Stomach.

6. Tilt: Do Lung Qi and Lung Yin descend to the Kidneys to enable the Kidneys to produce Kidney Yang and Kidney Yin? Simultaneously press the Lung and Spleen pulses down the tiniest amount and at the same time, release the tiniest amount of pressure from the Kidney pulse. The Kidney pulse should pop during the next beat.

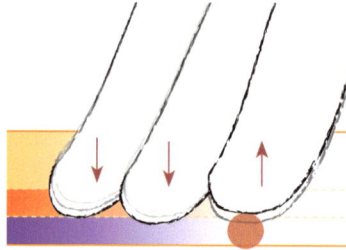

   a. If the Kidney pulse does pop we can say that Lung Qi does descend and is grasped by the Kidneys.

   b. If the Kidney pulse does not pop, we can say that the Lungs are not descending or that they are not descending optimally. A weakness in Kidney Yang could then be a false weakness (appearing to be weak when the Kidneys are not weak) since the Lungs are not nourishing the Kidneys.

   c. Note: You might feel that the Lung Qi descends under your fingers but not all the way to the Kidneys. The Kidneys are not popping because the Lung Qi is not reaching all the way to the Kidneys. Classically, Kidneys grasping Lung Qi was implied the complete descension of Lung Qi. In other words, if the descension of Lung Qi was complete, the Kidneys automatically received that Qi.

Note: The Stomach serves as an emissary for this action. If this vector is absent, it may mean that there is a blockage in the Middle Jiao.

7. Tilt (Advanced): Does Kidney Yang finance Wei Qi (at the Lung position) to enable the Lungs to perform their dispersing function? Press the Kidney pulse down the tiniest amount and almost immediately after that press the Spleen pulse down the tiniest amount and almost immediately after that, release the tiniest amount of pressure from the Lungs. The second pressure (the one at the Spleen) should palpably increase the hydraulic pressure moving up to the Lungs. The Lung pulse should give one pop during the next beat.

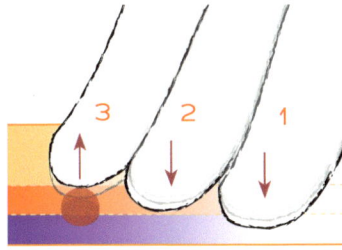

a. If the Lung pulse does pop we can say that Kidney Yang does finance Wei Qi.

b. During this advanced compound tilt you might notice a connection moving upward from the Kidney pulse to the Spleen pulse. Kidney Yang is supporting Spleen Yang. This leg of the pulse reflects the third trajectory of the Kidney Primary Channel which connects KI-2 to SP-8 and is the basis of digestive Qi.

8. Release: Does Heart Qi Disperse? Now, on the left wrist, much should be familiar already. As slowly as possible release pressure from the Heart pulse and allow your finger to follow the pulse upward toward the skin. The pulse should follow your finger much of the way to the skin level, and then scatter.

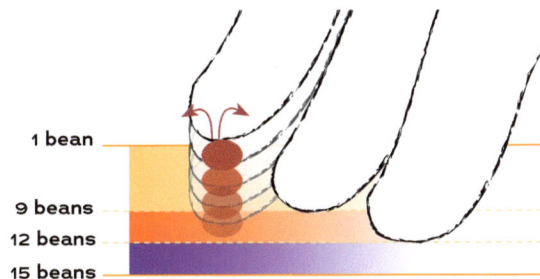

a. If the Heart pulse does follow your finger into the Wei level, we can say that the Heart is dispersing Qi.

b. If the Heart pulse does not follow your finger all the way to the surface, we can say that the Heart is not fully dispersing Qi.

9. Tilt: Do Liver Qi and Liver Blood ascend to engender Heart Qi and Heart Blood? Press the Liver pulse down the tiniest amount and at the same time, release the tiniest amount of pressure from the Heart pulse. The Heart pulse should give a pop during the next beat.

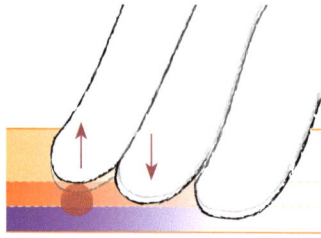

a. If the Heart pulse does pop we can say that Liver Blood does ascend to the Heart.

b. If the Heart pulse does not pop, we can say that the Liver is not ascending or that it is not ascending optimally.

10. Tilt: Does Liver Blood Descend to the Kidneys to nourish Kidney Yin?
    Press the Liver pulse down the tiniest amount and at the same time, release the tiniest amount of pressure from the Kidney pulse. The Kidney pulse should give a pop during the next beat.

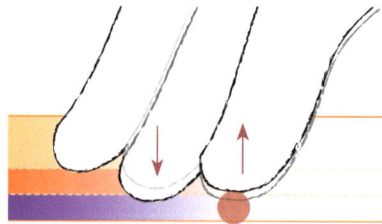

a. If the Kidney pulse does pop we can say that Liver Blood does nourish Kidney Yin.

b. If the Kidney pulse does not pop, we can say that Liver Blood is not descending to the Kidneys or that it is not descending optimally.

11. Tilt: Does the Heart communicate to the Kidneys?
    Press the Heart position and, almost immediately after that, press the Liver position down the tiniest amount, and almost immediately after that release the tiniest amount of pressure from the Kidney pulse. The Kidney pulse should give a pop during the next beat.

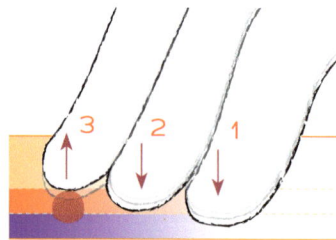

a. If the Kidney pulse does pop we can say that the Heart does communicate to the Kidneys.

b. If the Kidney pulse does not pop, we can say the communication of the Heart to the Kidneys is impeded somehow.

Note: The Liver serves as the emissary for this action. This means that in order for this communication to happen, the diaphragm must be free. A blockage in the Heart-Kidney vector may indicate a diaphragmatic blockage.

12. Tilt: Do the Kidneys communicate to the Heart? As the Kidneys contain Ancestral Qi—the repository of a person's destiny—and the Heart contains the individual's current experience of identity, reading the communication of Kidney to Heart essentially explores how well an individual is living his or her destiny. Traditionally, this pulse reading is considered to be intruding on the individual's sovereignty and is left unexplored, unread. This is beyond the role of the clinician/patient or even master/student relationship. The technique for reading this pulse, however, is no different from the others and is hypothetically explained here. Press the Kidney pulse down the tiniest amount and at the same time, release the tiniest amount of pressure from the Heart pulse. The Heart pulse should give one pop during the next beat.

a. If the Heart pulse does pop we can say that the Kidneys do communicate to the Heart.

b. If the Heart pulse does not pop, we can say the communication of the Kidneys to the Heart is impeded somehow.

SUMMARY OF DIRECTIONAL PULSE TAKING

Pressure must be maintained in all positions at all times.

1. *Assume pulse neutral position.*
2. *Release:* Are the Lungs capable of Dispersing? Release the Lung pulse.
3. *Tilt:* Does Spleen Qi ascend to the Lungs? Press both the Spleen and Kidney pulses down and release pressure from the Lung pulse.
4. *Release:* Is Triple Heater expressing something from the Jing? Is Kidney Yang escaping? Release pressure from the Kidney Yang pulse.
5. *Tilt:* Does Stomach Qi descend to the intestines? Press the Spleen pulse down and release the Kidney pulse.
6. *Tilt:* Do Lung Qi and Lung Yin descend to the Kidneys to enable the Kidneys to produce Kidney Yang and Kidney Yin? Press the Lung and Spleen pulses down

the tiniest amount and release the Kidney pulse.

7. *Tilt:* (Advanced) Does Kidney Yang finance Wei Qi (at the Lung position) to enable the Lungs to perform their dispersing function? Press the Kidney pulse down, then press the Spleen pulse down, then release pressure from the Lungs.

8. *Release:* Does Heart Qi Disperse? Release pressure from the Heart pulse.

9. *Tilt:* Do Liver Qi and Liver Blood ascend to engender Heart Qi and Heart Blood? Press the Liver pulse down and release pressure from the Heart pulse.

10. *Tilt:* Does Liver Blood Descend to the Kidneys to nourish Kidney Yin? Press the Liver pulse down and release pressure from the Kidney pulse.

11. *Tilt:* (Advanced) Does the Heart communicate to the Kidneys? Press the Heart pulse down, then the Liver position down, then release pressure from the Kidney pulse.

12. *Tilt:* Do the Kidneys communicate to the Heart? (If you choose to look.) Press the Kidney pulse down, then release the tiniest amount of pressure from the Heart pulse.

	R			L	
superficial	————			————	superficial
moderate	————	LU	HT	————	moderate
deep	————			————	deep
superficial	————			————	superficial
moderate	————	SP	LR	————	moderate
deep	————			————	deep
superficial	————			————	superficial
moderate	————	KI Yang	KI Yin	————	moderate
deep	————			————	deep

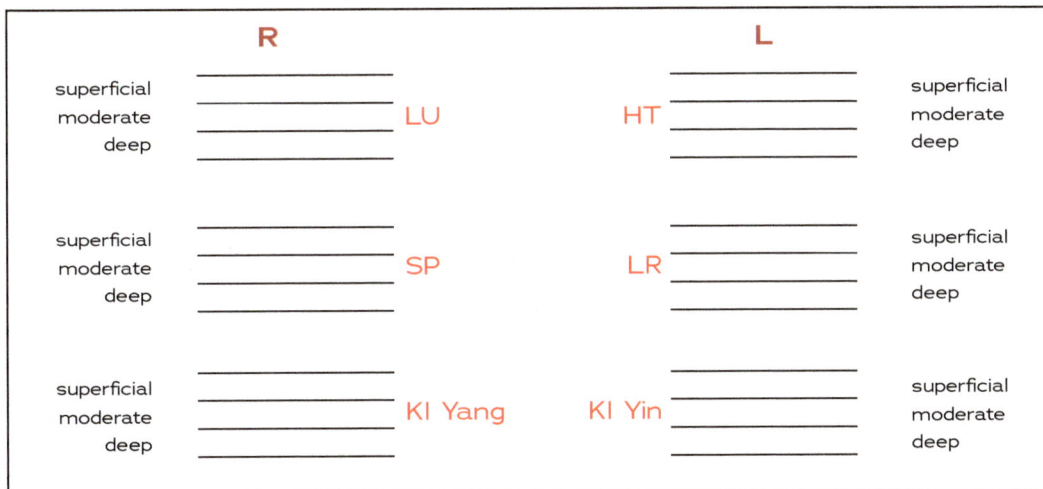

The three lines in each position are spaces for notating observations about the humors, Qi or Jin-Thin Fluids, Blood, Ye-Thick Fluids in each position.

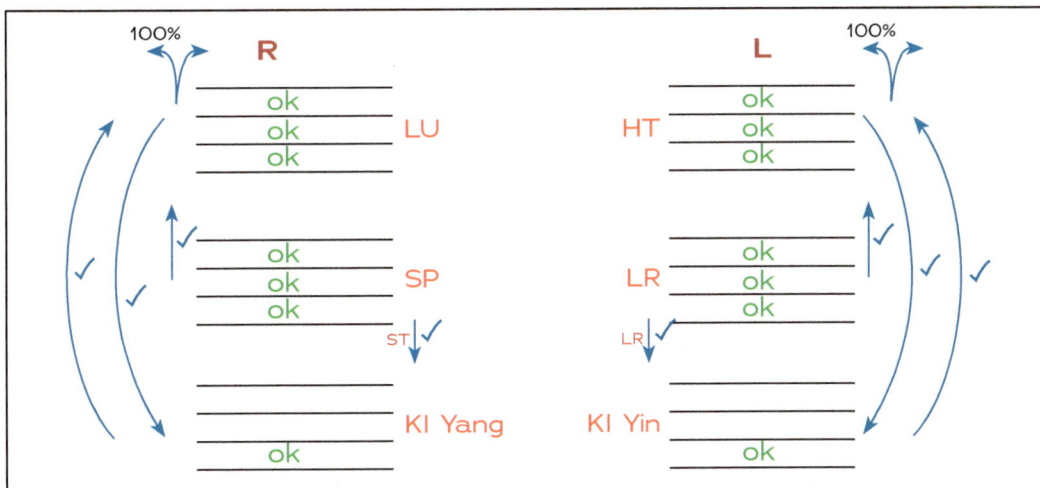

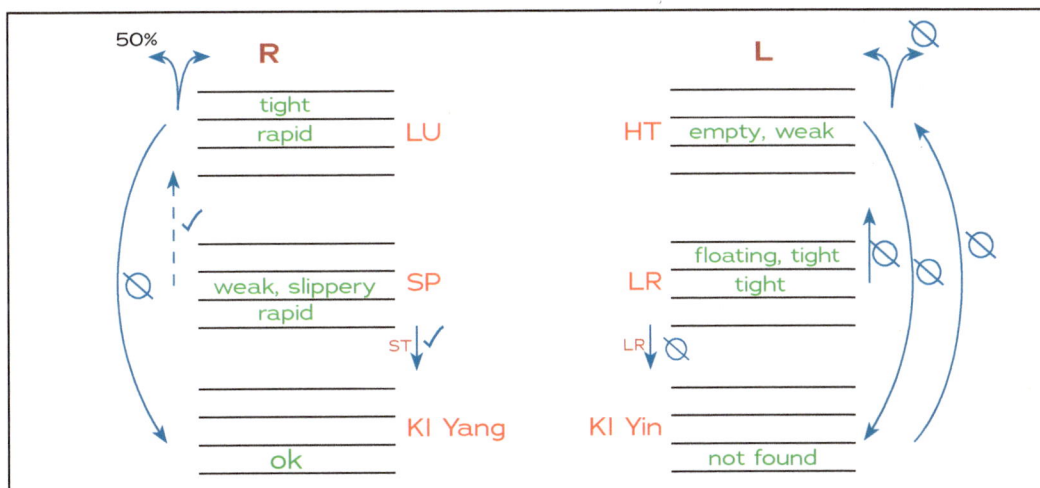

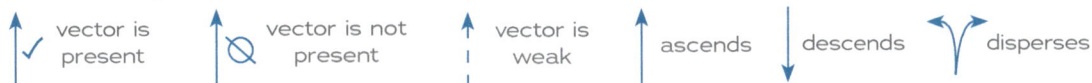

| vector is present | vector is not present | vector is weak | ascends | descends | disperses |

VERY BASIC TREATMENT OF DIRECTIONAL PULSE FINDINGS

Learning acupuncture is a long process in which acupuncture school is but a foundation. Point energetics are learned, then learned again, then learned in layers of historical meaning. Although points have function independently, point directionality and function are strongest in the context of a well-designed treatment. For example, BL-40 is sometimes taught as having the function of easing back pain, but that function is by far stronger and clearer when used in the context of a Bladder Divergent treatment. The acupuncturist gradually builds a personal knowledge of interwoven functionality of point energetics and associations.

AN EXAMPLE:

A patient complained of cough. The pulses show the Lungs were strong but that there was rebellious Stomach Qi. The Lungs were expressing the rebellion of the Stomach. A point that descends Lung Qi would not provide successful treatment. The treatment strategy must include descending the Stomach. There are many points that descend the Stomach, for example, ST-5 or ST-30. In this case CV-12 might best be chosen to perform this function since it is also the first point on the Lung Primary Channel.

Note: The list below comprises basic teaching examples only. There are countless ways to correct and generate these vectors using knowledge of point function. The correct approach will vary from patient to patient according to their strengths and weaknesses and their accompanying signs and symptoms.

1. *Lung dispersal.* To disperse the Lungs, choose a point with that function. For example, LU-1, LU-7 or LU-8 disperse the Lungs.

2. *Spleen to Lung ascension.* KI-2, SP-8, and LU-1 together ascend Spleen Qi to the Lungs.

3. *Kidney Yang is escaping or Triple Heater releases toxins.* Nourishing Yin enables Yang to be anchored. Bleeding GB-36 releases toxicity from the Yuan level. (If practicing the Complement Channels, Triple Heater Divergent Channel needled deep-superficial-deep returns toxicity to the Yuan level for later expulsion.)

4. *Stomach descension.* ST-5, CV-12 and ST-30 descend the Stomach, for example.

5. *Lung Qi and Lung Yin descension to the Kidneys.* Choose a point that descends Lung Qi, for example, LU-5. Connecting the water point of the Lungs and the metal point of the Kidneys would be one way to create this descension.

6. *Kidney Yang generating Wei Qi.* Usually ascension of Kidney Yang generates stimulation of this vector as long as blockages are not in play. KI-2 to SP-8 ascends Kidney Yang to the Spleen and LU-1 takes it up to the Lungs. (See Inter-Jiao Blockages, p. 87.)

7. *Liver ascension to Heart.* I usually use a whole channel to create this vector, such as Yin Wei Mai or Liver Divergent, but as points, LR-14 and CV-14 needled with intention to connect, create this vector. The second branch of the Liver Primary Channel also makes this vector: LR-14, CV-12, PC-1.

8. *Heart dispersal.* This vector seems only to appear if the patient feels connection to humanity or if the person has optimism, which perhaps only exist in parallel. The practitioner's optimism and open heart create this vector.

9. *Liver descension.* LR-14 can produce this vector. Yin Wei Mai produces this vector.

10. *Heart to Kidney communication and Kidney to Heart communication.* I usually use whole channels such as Chong or Yin Wei Mai to create these vectors. KI-21 creates these vectors on its own, however.

INTER-JIAO BLOCKAGES: THE DIAPHRAGM AND DAI MAI

Inter-Jiao blockages can prevent the free flow of Qi from one organ to another. The most common external cause of these blockages is Cold. Emotions are the most common internal cause. Ultimately, if untreated, blockages affect the entire system as the movement of Qi is progressively impeded. Blockages can prevent the success of any treatment and must be released. Fortunately, the technique of Directional pulses enables the practitioner to find blockages relatively easily.

Inter-Jiao blockages should not be confused with tightness. Very often, tight pulses indicate a positive response in the body to a lack of some kind of mediumship (Fluids, Blood, Yin). For example, if the Liver pulse is tight, it's likely that there is a Blood deficiency and the body is trying to hold onto Blood. Releasing this tightness can result in prolonging the Blood deficiency as the body gathers more Qi to reinstate the tightness in order to place Blood in reserve. It's essential to separate pathological tightness from tightness generated by the body as a response to pathology. Tightness generated as a response to pathology is not pathology itself. In the case above, the nourishment of Blood would result in the Liver relaxing. That is, the tight response to the pathology of Blood deficiency falls away when Blood deficiency is resolved.

Inter-Jiao blockages can cause an organ to appear deficient when it is not. For example, the Lungs might appear weak, but that may be an illusion; they may simply not be receiving Qi from the Spleen because the diaphragm is blocking it. (Qi from a weak or tight Spleen might not reach the Lungs either.) Tonifying Lung Qi would not yield lasting results, or no result at all, but if the lack of communication is due to a blockage of the diaphragm, releasing that blockage in the diaphragm would enable the Lungs to act in their full capacity. The Lungs could also appear weak if Kidney Yang is not reaching the Spleen. This could show as tightness in Kidney Yang, a Yang deficiency, a blockage in the low back, or a blockage in Dai Mai. Tonifying Lung Qi or Spleen Qi would yield no positive result in the Lungs, but treating the Kidneys or the blockage in Dai Mai would.

Diaphragmatic blockages are likely present if:
- on both wrists the guan positions do not communicate up to the cun positions.
- while performing any of the described tilt actions to or from the cun position, the position being pressed becomes stronger and the receiving pulse does not react. For example, when checking that the Spleen is able to ascend its Qi to the Lungs (pressing the guan position down and releasing the Lung position) the Spleen pulse surges but the Lung pulse does not respond at all, a blockage is present in the diaphragm.
- there is a palpable bulge between the cun and the guan positions.

Dai Mai blockage is likely present if:
- on both wrists the guan positions do not communicate down to the chi positions.
- while performing any of the described tilt actions to or from the chi position, the position being pressed becomes stronger and the receiving pulse does not react. For example, when checking that the Liver is able to descend its Qi to the Kidneys (pressing the guan position down and releasing the Kidney position) the Liver pulse surges but the Kidney pulse does not respond at all, a blockage is present in Dai Mai.
- there is a palpable bulge between the cun and the guan positions.

TREATMENT OF INTER-JIAO BLOCKAGES

There are limitless options for releasing inter-Jiao blockages. Choose points with which you resonate. These are the ones I resonate with in case it's helpful.

To release the diaphragm: release LR-14. Insert very obliquely, reduce strongly and remove. Or release LR-13 in a similar way. Or reduce LR-6 and LU-6. Or reduce BL-17 at the Hua To position.

To release Dai Mai, needle GB-41, GB-26, GB-27 and GB-28 unilaterally (left in males, right in females) and vibrate until the patient feels a very subtle descending feeling in the lower abdomen.

To further release blockages, consider releasing a tight pulse by reducing the Mu point of the related organ.

It is, of course, essential to release any Sinew pulse (any tight, superficial pulse). The method chosen could involve sliding cups or gua sha on the Sinew Channel indicated, a full Sinew treatment, or the release of the Jing-Well point of the channel indicated. Most of these releases take a few minutes.

Check the pulses to ensure the blockage has been released before proceeding with the remainder of the treatment. If the blockage has been cleared:
• either or both of the guan positions will freely communicate up to the cun or down to the chi.
• a pulse will not become fuller when it is pressed during a tilt action.
• bulges between the guan and either the cun or chi will no longer be present.

REFUSAL
Refusal in the pulses means the healthy circulation of Qi is interrupted not by deficiency nor by blockage, but because the receiving organ for some reason is not receptive to the Qi that nourishes it. The possibility of a blockage should be eliminated before considering refusal. The tendency of an organ to refuse Qi or mediumship can be determined while taking of directional pulses. For example, while using the Tilt action to determine whether the Lungs are able to receive Qi from the Spleen, if you find that the Spleen pulse becomes fuller (instead of the Lung pulse, which we would expect) the Lungs are said to be refusing Spleen Qi. The organ refusing Qi can do so in order to protect an emotional status quo. For example, the Lungs can refuse Qi if there is a conscious or unconscious desire to suppress grief. The added Qi would perhaps stimulate the Lungs to express the grief, but the patient is not ready or unwilling to process it.

REFUSAL IN THE KIDNEY YANG POSITION
If the Kidneys refuse blood from the Heart it is said that the Pericardium is active in defending the Heart. This is confirmed by examining both wrists at the same time. A pulse will emerge in the moderate level of the Kidney Yang position and there can be a tightening at the Heart position at the same time. If, conversely, the Heart refuses Blood the patient is not ready to look at emotional issues. This, of course, should be respected.

FAILURE TO RECEIVE

Failure to receive is also determined during directional pulse taking. If, while using the Tilt action, Qi or Fluid is felt moving toward the receiving organ but the receiving organ does not accept it, the receiving organ is said to fail to receive. This is sometimes felt while determining communication between Lungs and Kidneys when Qi is felt leaving the Lung position but does not cause a reaction (pop) in the Kidney position. In this case, the Lungs are descending Qi but the Kidneys are not receiving (grasping) it. An organ might not receive Qi if it is lacking the Yang Qi to hold the incoming medium in place. It might also not receive Qi in order to maintain a convenient emotional status quo. For example, in patients who are reluctant to enter into what they feel is their true path, the Heart might not receive communication from the Kidneys because to do so would raise awareness of their destiny and the responsibility to live it. If the Heart doesn't receive Blood, recommend the patient stop all hot spices, garlic and coffee; the Heart may be occupied scattering Heat.

REFUSAL VERSUS FAILURE TO RECEIVE

Refusal and failure to receive differ in that during refusal the destination organ pushes the delivery back at the organ of origin (the sender), causing pulse of the organ of origin to swell momentarily. Failure to receive implies the receiving organ would be happy to accept delivery if it had the means to hold onto it.

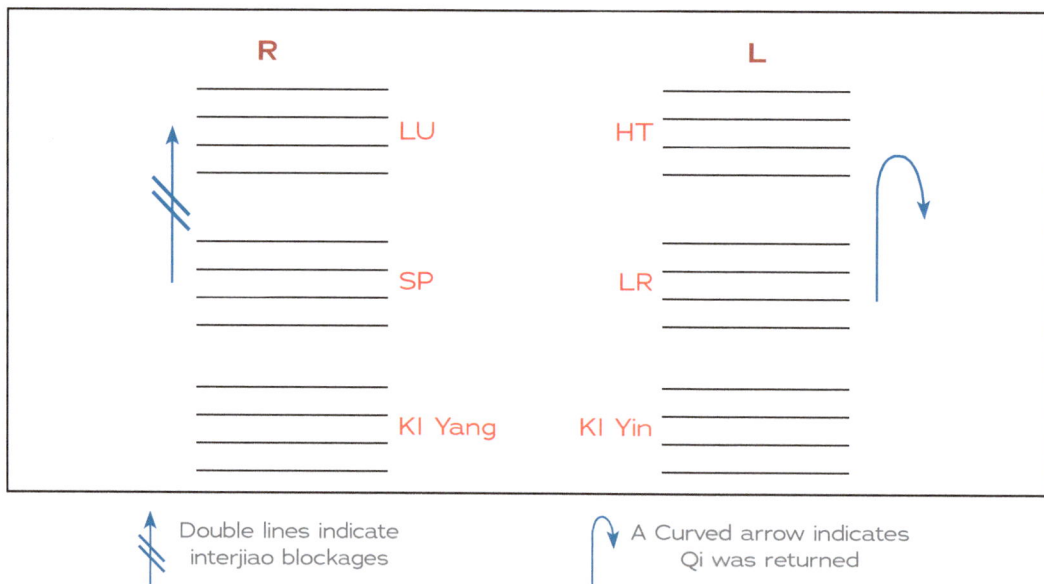

Double lines indicate interjiao blockages

A Curved arrow indicates Qi was returned

About the Author

Ann Cecil-Sterman, MS, L.Ac, is the author of the widely acclaimed book, *Advanced Acupuncture: A Clinic Manual*, a required text in many acupuncture schools in the United States. She travels all over the world to teach the application and methodology of the Complement Channels, the art of pulse diagnosis, and the use of food as medicine. For many years she taught Advanced Clinical Observation and was a senior clinic supervisor at the school of acupuncture founded by Dr Jeffrey Yuen in 1997 in New York City. She is a long-time student of Dr Yuen, having extensively studied acupuncture, diet, Chinese medical history, herbs, qigong, essential oils, stones and philosophy with him across North America. She also studied pulses and the Complementary Channels with Dr Sheila George. Ann was Director of the Classical Wellness Center in Manhattan where for many yeats she practiced and taught classes on advanced diagnosis and the theory and application of Classical Chinese Medicine. Currently, her patients—children and adults of all ages— come from all over the world, working through illnesses or on personal cultivation. Ann's practice features the Complement Channels of acupuncture: the Sinew, Luo, Divergent and Eight Extraordinary Channels, and is augmented with Classical Chinese dietary therapeutic guidance. She lives in Manhattan with her husband and two children.

About the Illustrator

Cody Dodo, MS, L.Ac, studied acupuncture under the tutelage of Dr Jeffery Yuen at the Swedish Institute in New York. He also completed advanced studies with Dr Yuen in acupuncture and Chinese nutritional therapy. He lectures about Chinese Medicine in New York, and internationally. Prior to his pursuit of acupuncture, Cody had a long career as a graphic designer in the publishing industry. By combining his Chinese medical knowledge with his visual sensibility, Cody is able to convey the author's ideas with clear and simple diagrams and design. He also designed the Author's first book, *Advanced Acupuncture: A Clinic Manual.* He has a private practice in Manhattan, and lives with his wife in Brooklyn.

By the Same Author

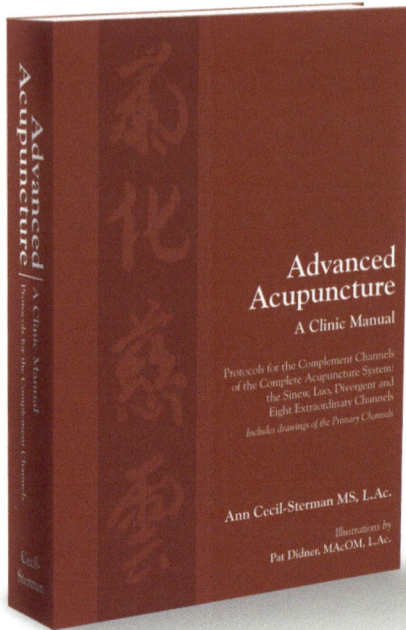

Advanced Acupuncture, A Clinic Manual
Protocols for the Complement Channels of the
Complete Acupuncture System: the Sinew, Luo, Divergent
and Eight Extraordinary Channels

Classical Wellness Press, 2012

Currently a required or recommended text in many acupuncture schools.

Illustrations of the Complete Acupuncture System:
the Sinew, Luo, Divergent, Eight Extraordinary
and Primary Channels

Classical Wellness Press, 2014.

(This is a companion volume to _Advanced Acupuncture, A Clinic Manual_
and is not a stand-alone book. It's designed to make the Manual's
illustrations easily accessible in ring-bound form.)

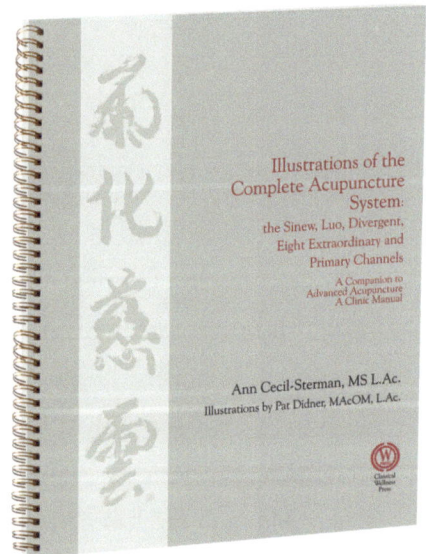